Ageless Nutrition and Fitness

Stay Fit and Healthy Over 50

Table of Contents

Chapter 1. Introduction

Welcome to the vibrant journey of 'Ageless Nutrition and Fitness: Stay Fit and Healthy Over 50'! In this remarkable Special Report, we unveil the secrets to maintaining a robust and radiant life after 50. As we age, our bodies undergo changes requiring special care and attention, particularly concerning nutrition and fitness. But who says this has to be daunting or confusing? Certainly, not this report! With a zestful approach, insightful guidance, and easy-to-follow tips, we're here to show you how to enjoy the golden years with gusto! This report does not just focus on longevity, but rather, the journey to ensure that these years are filled with joy, energy, and vitality. Excited? So are we! Let's defy age together and pave a road that will lead you to a healthful life, bursting with well-being. Your quest for joyous aging starts here!

Chapter 2. Understanding the Aging Process: Nutrition and Fitness

Let's start by understanding what happens as we age. Aging is a natural process that we all experience - it's a complex process characterized by a progressive decline in physiological functions, which, in turn, increases the risk of disease and death. However, the rate at which we age varies from individual to individual and is influenced by factors such as genetics, lifestyle, and environmental elements.

2.1. Physiological Changes as We Age

While some people remain healthy into their eighties and beyond, others may face health issues earlier due to several changes that occur in our bodies as we age.

Loss of Muscle Mass: Also known as sarcopenia, loss of muscle mass occurs naturally from the age of 50, with a more profound decline after the age of 60. This occurs because of hormonal changes, a decrease in physical activity, and loss of nerve cells that send signals to the muscles to move.

Reduced Metabolic Rate: Simple tasks such as breathing, digesting food, or repairing cells all require energy, and the total amount of energy our bodies use to carry out these fundamental functions is known as our metabolic rate. As we age, our metabolic rate decreases, which can lead to weight gain if diet and exercise aren't adjusted accordingly.

Dehydrated Skin: Human skin comprises mostly water. As we age, aging skin tends to be thinner, less elastic, and drier. This can create wrinkles, deep lines, and a pale, sagging appearance.

2.2. Nutritional Needs for Older Adults

Our nutritional needs change as we get older. Consuming a nutritious diet becomes even more critical for staying healthy, maintaining muscle mass, promoting a healthy immune system, and supporting cognitive health.

Protein: Higher intake of dietary protein is associated with a reduced risk of frailty. Active people over the age of 50 should aim to consume around 1 to 1.2 grams of protein per kilogram of body weight.

Calcium and Vitamin D: Calcium and Vitamin D support bone health. The intake of these nutrients may mitigate the natural loss of bone density that happens with aging.

Omega-3 fatty acids: These essential fats can reduce inflammation in the body, which is linked to a range of chronic diseases.

Vitamins B12 and Folate: Both nutrients are crucial for the nervous system and maintaining good brain health.

2.3. Fitness and Aging

Regular physical activity improves health and can delay the aging process. It's beneficial for maintaining physical strength, keeping a healthy body weight, and improving balance, all of which reduces the risk of falls and injuries.

Aerobic Exercise: Activities such as brisk walking, cycling, or swimming can help to maintain a healthy heart and lungs.

Resistance Exercise: Activities such as weight lifting or resistance band exercises can help to maintain muscle mass and strength, which naturally decrease with age.

Flexibility Exercise: Activities such as yoga or Pilates can help maintain flexibility and range of movement, both of which can significantly aid in daily activities as we age.

Balance Exercise: Balance training can be beneficial for older adults to help prevent falls and sustain independence.

2.4. Staying Motivated for Fitness

Finding a routine and sticking to it can be challenging for anyone. But finding a fitness routine that you enjoy, that suits your ability, and that fits into your lifestyle is critical. Remain flexible, listen to your body and adapt as necessary. Celebrate small victories and give yourself credit when credit is due.

2.5. Your Mind-Body Connection

Aging without vitality is merely survival. Your mental wellbeing is just as crucial as your physical condition towards ensuring healthy aging. Two ways you can do this is through maintaining a positive mindset and staying socially engaged.

Positive Mindset: A positive mindset can enhance immune function, increase longevity, prevent chronic disease, and reduce stress levels.

Social Engagement: Sustaining social ties can reduce the risk of disability, increase longevity, and improve mental health. Activities such as group fitness classes, volunteering, or joining a club can help you stay connected.

Understanding the aging process, the role of nutrition, and the importance of fitness can greatly enhance our golden years. Armed with this knowledge, it's easier to make informed decisions, nurture our bodies, and live vibrantly. Your future self will thank you for taking these proactive steps today!

Chapter 3. Redefining Diet: Healthy Eating Habits for the Aged

As we cross the age threshold of fifty, our bodies undergo transformation. Nutrition absorption rates shift, metabolism tends to slow down, and our physiological needs evolve. By understanding these changes and adjusting our diet and nutrition plans accordingly, we can live the ageless life of health and vitality we all desire.

3.1. Understanding Dietary Changes with Age

Chalk and cheese, fire and ice, or oil and water — whatever metaphor you choose, the nutritional needs of a 30-year-old and a 50-year-old are as different as two things can be. Our bodies change as we age. This involves, among other aspects, a decrease in metabolism, changes in the digestive system, and an increased need for certain nutrients. Let's take these one at a time.

Metabolism naturally slows down with age. This is the primary reason why an older person may struggle with weight gain even when consuming the same diet as their younger self. The digestive system also goes through changes with a decrease in the secretion of digestive enzymes, which can lead to problems in absorption of vitamins and minerals.

In response to these changes, the need for certain nutrients increases. Calcium and Vitamin D are among these, needed in higher amounts to maintain bone health. Similarly, B-vitamins become more crucial as absorption rates decrease.

3.2. Staying Active: Tuning Up Metabolism

Remember this: age doesn't have to translate into a slower metabolism. While it is true that metabolism tends to decrease as we age, it is not set in stone. By staying physically active, we can maintain a healthy metabolism, which aids in maintaining a healthy weight and vigor. Physical activity also increases the absorption of nutrients from food, helping stave off nutritional deficiencies.

Starting with a simple routine, such as a daily walk, garden work, or gentle yoga, can kick-start your journey towards an active lifestyle. However, keep in mind that individual limitations may apply, so consult with a healthcare professional before starting a new exercise routine.

3.3. Building a Balanced Diet: The Ingredients

An age-friendly diet relies on quality over quantity, emphasizing nutrient-rich foods over calorie-dense but nutritionally poor choices. Choose whole grain foods for carbohydrates, lean sources of protein, and plenty of fruits and vegetables. Opt for 'good fats' over 'bad fats' – this means avocados and olive oil over trans fats and fried foods.

Dairy products or alternatives (like almond milk or soy milk) are recommended for their high calcium content. A variety of nuts and seeds, as well as oily fish, can provide the necessary Omega-3 fatty acids.

For Vitamin B, turn to whole grains, eggs, nuts, and dairy products. Do note, you may choose to take vitamin supplements, but it's always best to consult a healthcare provider first.

3.4. Hydration: Often Overlooked but Crucial

Staying hydrated is critical at all ages but is often overlooked, particularly in the older population. As we age, our sense of thirst diminishes, and we may not drink enough water. Besides, certain medications may cause dehydration.

Make a habit of drinking water throughout the day, even if you don't feel thirsty. Juices, soups, and specifically water-rich fruits and vegetables, such as cucumbers, can also contribute to hydration levels.

3.5. Smart Eating Habits

Diet is not only about what we eat, but also how and when we eat. Small and frequent meals are generally recommended, as they are easier to digest and help maintain stable blood sugar levels.

Not to forget, mealtimes should be a joy. Eating is not just physical nourishment; it is a sensory and social experience. Attending to the taste, texture, and aroma of the food we consume, eating with loved ones – all this creates a nurturing eating environment aiding digestion and nutrient absorption.

In conclusion, reaching the golden age of 50 is no reason to step back in life. With smart dietary practices, increased physical activity, and the right attitude, these can be, indeed, your most vibrant, active, and joyous years. The key lies in being informed about your changing nutritional needs, eating a varied and balanced diet, staying hydrated, and maintaining active lifestyle habits.

Remember, 'aging' is not just a biological process but a journey that can be steered in the direction of health, fitness, and joy. So, cheers to many more years of radiant health and vitality! After all, age is but a number when you have the right tips at your fingertips!

Chapter 4. Unlocking the Potential of Exercise for the Over 50s

Whether you are newly over 50 or have had a few years to acclimate to this age group, one thing is for sure: Exercise is an essential component of your health and well-being. Now more than ever, staying active is vital as it provides countless benefits, from physical conditioning and improved energy to cognitive function preservation and emotional health. For this reason, we have dedicated a considerable amount of time and resources to unpack every aspect of exercise for this important demographic. From which activities to go for to how to get started safely, everything you need to know about exercise for the over 50s is right here. So, let's get down to details.

4.1. Understanding the Benefits of Exercise

While most of us have a general idea that staying active is good for us, it is essential to understand how prevalent this is, particularly for individuals over 50. Regular physical activity is, in fact, a strong weapon against many health problems common in this age group.

To start with, it drastically reduces the risk of various diseases, including heart disease, stroke, type 2 diabetes, and certain types of cancers. Since these diseases are more prevalent in people over 50, your benefit from regular physical activity is even greater. Moreover, exercise promotes weight management and healthy bone density, reducing the risk of osteoporosis, another common concern for those over 50.

Cognitive health also experiences a boost, thanks to regular physical activity. Exercise aids in maintaining good blood flow to the brain, and through its effect on hormones, it helps foster new brain cell growth and preservation of existing cells.

In terms of emotional health, being active helps ward off depression and decreases anxiety levels while improving overall mood. The latter is often linked with a better quality of sleep, another essential aspect of good health as we age.

What's more, exercise even helps with controlling chronic pain and improving flexibility and mobility, leading to better balance and reducing the risk of falls.

4.2. Choosing Age-Appropriate Activities

While understanding the importance of exercise is the first step, figuring out what type of activities are most beneficial can be a bit more complex. Exercises can basically be divided into four types – endurance, strength, balance, and flexibility. As an individual over 50, your routine should ideally be a mix of all these types of activities.

Endurance or aerobic exercises, like brisk walking, swimming, or cycling, are essential to maintain a healthy heart and circulatory system. For strength training, activities such as weight lifting or resistance band exercises help keep muscles strong, which is incredibly important as muscle mass tends to decrease with age.

Flexibility exercises, such as stretching and yoga, play a crucial role in maintaining mobility, while balance exercises are vital in preventing falls – a common issue for older people.

4.3. Starting Safely

Despite the numerous benefits, it's essential to remember that safety should always come first, especially when you begin a new exercise regimen. If you've been inactive for a while, start with light activities and gradually increase intensity and duration.

A crucial aspect of safety is awareness of your body. Learning to differentiate between good and bad pain, knowing when to push and when to step back is vital to prevent injuries. Further, you should always warm up before exercising and cool down after to avoid muscle strains.

4.4. Overcoming Common Barriers

Despite the importance of regular exercise, starting and maintaining a consistent workout program can be a considerable challenge, especially for people over 50. Physical discomfort, lack of time, and low motivation are common barriers.

Remember that any movement is better than none. Even if you can't follow a traditional workout routine, you can still reap the benefits of activity. It may involve walking instead of driving, doing some light gardening, or choosing stairs over the elevator.

4.5. Monitoring Your Progress

Lastly, it's important to continuously monitor your progress. Whether it's walking for a few more minutes, lifting heavier weights, or mastering a new yoga pose, celebrating progress can be a powerful form of motivation.

Remember, it's never too late to start. Incorporating regular exercise into your daily routine may seem challenging at first, but the benefits are immense. After a while, you will wonder how you ever did without it!

So, why not start today? Your healthier, fitter self awaits you. No matter what your age is, you have the power to change, to grow, to improve. Embrace it! Allow exercise to not merely add years to your life, but life to your years.

Chapter 5. The Role of Hydration in Ageless Health

Understanding our body's complex mechanisms can seem like a daunting task. However, it is essential towards enhancing our well-being. A vital element that might seem overly simple but holds immense importance in our overall health is water. Our bodies are approximately 60% water, and this ratio is slightly higher in older age. Let's delve deeper into understanding the crucial role that hydration plays in maintaining ageless health.

5.1. The Importance of Staying Hydrated

The human body is mostly composed of water, and it is strongly tied to our overall functioning. Our brains depend on proper hydration to function optimally, along with critical body functions such as nutrient transport, body temperature regulation, and waste management. When our bodies lack water, these functions can deteriorate, increasing the risk of health issues.

Make no mistake: all cells, tissues, and organs in our bodies need water. From maintaining the health of our skin to ensuring the proper functioning of our kidneys and maintaining our cognitive performance, water is indispensable. Additionally, water acts as a lubricant for our joints, preventing the wear and tear that leads to painful conditions like arthritis.

5.2. Hydration and Aging

As we age, our body composition changes, leading to lesser water content in our bodies. Furthermore, our sense of thirst also diminishes over time, meaning older adults may not drink water even if they are dehydrated. Along with this, many medications that older individuals take can also lead to increased fluid loss, further accentuating the problem.

In older adults, even mild dehydration can lead to severe health problems like urinary tract infections, confusion, and an increased risk of falls. Proper hydration, on the other hand, aids digestion, absorption, and transportation of nutrients, promoting optimal health.

5.3. Guidelines for Hydration

While the old adage of drinking eight glasses of water a day is a useful measure; individual requirements vary widely. Factors such as your diet, physical activity levels, and the local climate all influence your hydration needs. As a thumb rule, you should aim for a minimum of 1.5 liters of water per day, with an increase during times of increased physical activity, or hot weather.

But plain water isn't the only way to stay hydrated. Other beverages such as herbal teas, milk, and clear broths also contribute to hydration. Furthermore, many fruits and vegetables have high water content and can aid in maintaining an optimal hydration level.

Remember, some beverages work against hydration. Alcoholic and caffeinated drinks can cause fluid loss, and sugary drinks lead to unnecessary calorie intake. Consumption of these should be kept to a moderate level.

5.4. Monitor Your Hydration Levels

Keeping an eye on your hydration level is as important as ingesting an adequate amount of fluids daily. One of the simplest ways to check if you're adequately hydrated is through the color of your urine.

Light straw or pale yellow urine typically indicates proper hydration, while darker urine can be a sign of dehydration.

Apart from this, frequently feeling thirsty, experiencing a dry mouth, tiredness, headache, and reduced urine output can also signal inadequate hydration. It is essential always to take these signs seriously and act promptly to restore your body's hydration balance.

5.5. The Role of Diet in Hydration

A balanced diet can significantly assist in maintaining good hydration levels. Foods with high water content, like cucumbers, watermelon, oranges, and strawberries, can supplement your daily fluid intake. Salads, broths, and soups also carry substantial amounts of water, apart from being rich in essential nutrients.

5.6. The Role of Exercise in Hydration

Physical activity invariably increases sweat production, thus leading to fluid loss. It's crucial to balance this loss by consuming enough fluids before, during, and after exercise to prevent dehydration. Moreover, exercising individuals should be watchful of symptoms like dizziness, dry mouth, fatigue, and low urine output, as they can be signs of dehydration.

5.7. Hydration and Chronic Conditions

Certain chronic health conditions like diabetes, kidney disease, heart failure, and certain neurological conditions might change how your body regulates fluids. In such cases, being mindful of hydration levels is critical. Having conversations with your healthcare provider about how much water you should drink can be extremely useful in these scenarios.

In conclusion, hydration is an essential aspect of overall health and wellness, especially as we age. Lack of appropriate hydration can lead to varied health issues while maintaining good hydration levels can boost vitality, enhance physical and cognitive performance, and drastically improve the quality of life. Therefore, it's crucial to be mindful of your hydration status, supplementing it with a balanced diet, and resorting to corrective actions when showing signs of dehydration. After all, age is just a number, and with proper hydration, the journey towards healthful and joyous aging takes on a smoother, easier ride.

Chapter 6. Boosting Immunity: Superfoods for the 50s and Beyond

A robust immune system is your body's battle line defense against various illnesses and diseases. As we hit the marks of 50 and above, our immune system experiences a decline. However, though this is a normal part of aging, it doesn't mean we can't boost our immune functions. In this chapter, we'll explore the potent power of superfoods and how these dietary heavyweights can reinforce your immune system and maintain your overall health.

6.1. Nurturing the Immune System

The health of your immune system heavily correlates with what you eat. Adopting a proper diet means providing your immune cells with the nutrients they need to function effectively. Superfoods, packed with essential vitamins, minerals, fiber, and antioxidants, contribute to a resilient immune system. Consuming a diet rich with these nutrient-dense foods improves digestion, reduces inflammation, and optimizes your body's natural defenses.

6.2. Eating the Rainbow

Governed by the principle "Eating the Rainbow," including a variety of colored fruits and vegetables in your diet is a step towards a supercharged immune system. Each color signifies different nutrient profiles, providing a range of antioxidants your body can benefit from.

- **Red fruits and vegetables** like tomatoes and strawberries are rich in antioxidants such as lycopene and Vitamin C.

- **Orange and yellow** items like carrots and oranges pack a punch of carotenoids including Vitamin A, important for a strong immune system.

- **Green foods** like spinach and kale contain numerous nutrients, including Vitamins C and E and folate.

- **Blue and purple foods** such as blueberries and eggplants are high in anthocyanins. Anthocyanins are powerful antioxidants that help enhance immunity.

6.3. Superfoods to Include in Your Diet

There are numerous superfoods you can incorporate into your diet to boost your immune system. Let us break these down.

- **Citrus fruits**: Source of Vitamin C, which aids in the production of white blood cells - the defenders of our body.

- **Almonds**: Rich in Vitamin E, crucial for maintaining a healthy immune system, particularly in older adults.

- **Broccoli**: Packed with Vitamins C, A, and E, fiber and many other antioxidants.

- **Green tea**: Contains flavonoids and L-theanine which may aid in the production of germ-fighting compounds in your T-cells.

- **Spinach**: Rich in Vitamin C and packed with numerous antioxidants and beta carotene.

- **Turmeric**: Known for its anti-inflammatory effects, it can also enhance immune responses.

- **Yogurt**: Great source of probiotics which enhances the gut health, leading towards a stronger immune system.

- **Garlic**: Helps boost immune cell function and may also have anti-inflammatory properties.

- **Papaya**: Packed with Vitamin C, digestive enzymes, and a decent amount of folate and potassium.

6.4. Planning a Superfood-Rich Diet

Generating a diet plan rich in superfoods may feel overwhelming, but with thoughtful meal planning, it can be simple and enjoyable.

Breakfast: Start your day with a green tea, followed by a bowl of Greek yogurt enriched with almonds and fruits like papaya or berries.

Lunch: Prepare a colourful salad with veggies like spinach, tomatoes, and bell peppers topped with olive oil and garlic dressing.

Dinner: A warm bowl of lean meat or tofu stew with turmeric, carrots, broccoli, and other veggies is a good option.

Snacks: Granola bars, citrus fruit salads, or simple almonds can fit the bill.

6.5. Consistency is Key

While incorporating these superfoods into your diet, remember that consistency is the key. Training your palate to enjoy these superfoods isn't always an easy journey, but the fruits reaped— stronger immunity and improved overall health — are absolutely worthwhile.

6.6. Superfoods and Holistic Health

No singular superfood guarantees immunity, nor can one dietary change cause drastic improvements overnight. However, a nutritious diet forms the bedrock for overall health and improved immunity. Remember to accompany your superfood-rich diet with a balanced lifestyle that incorporates ample sleep, regular exercise, and minimal stress.

6.7. Seeking Professional Advice

Before passionately diving into any drastic dietary changes, consulting a medical professional, or a certified dietitian is highly recommended, especially for individuals with specific dietary restrictions or chronic conditions.

In conclusion, boosting your immunity through diet requires more than just having an apple a day to keep the doctor away. A proactive approach to nutrition, focusing on a variety of superfoods, consistency, and balanced lifestyle choices, can genuinely lead you towards a healthier life post 50. Let's take the next step in our aging journey proactively and deliciously. Let's keep our immunity strong and bodies resilient with the power of superfoods. After all, we're in this vibrantly engaging journey together!

Chapter 7. The Power of Mind-Body Connection: Yoga and Meditation

As we journey into the age of 50 and beyond, we often realize the indispensable role of mindfulness in our journey toward holistic wellness. By focusing our energies on harmonizing the mind and body, we can not only mitigate age-related ailments but also procure a serene sense of inner peace. The tools we're going to explore in this context are Yoga and Meditation, potent instruments in forging and fortifying this crucial mind-body connection.

7.1. Understanding the Mind-Body Connection

The mind-body connection is not a new concept; it has roots in ancient philosophies and medical systems, such as Ayurveda and Traditional Chinese Medicine. Modern science, too, acknowledges this intrinsic link, witnessing the interplay between psychological processes and bodily functions. Simply put, our emotional, mental, social, and spiritual states can directly affect our physical health.

For aging individuals, harnessing this mind-body connection is paramount. With progressive years come greater complexities in health, reflecting in forms such as chronic diseases, decreased physical strength, and cognitive decline. This is where our practices–Yoga and Meditation, imbued with the energy of mindfulness and bodily harmonization, become central to aging healthily.

7.2. Yoga: The Journey of Self-Discovery

Touted as the 'universal practical school of self-realization', Yoga goes beyond mere physical exercise. It is meditative, spiritual, and deeply transformative, enabling individuals to connect with their inner selves while promoting physical well-being.

7.2.1. Yoga for Physical Well-Being

As we age, maintaining physical strength and flexibility takes precedence. Regular Yoga practices can play an instrumental role in this regard, fostering performances in daily activities and decelerating the aging process.

Various forms of Yoga postures or 'asanas' aid in improving our balance control, flexibility, and muscular strength. They offer a low-impact yet effective alternative to vigorous exercises, making it suitable for older adults.

7.2.2. Yoga for Mental Peace

Beyond the physical realm, Yoga has profound effects on our mental health. It helps to mitigate stress, tension, and anxiety, which are common as we navigate the intricacies of life past 50. 'Pranayama', the yogic practice of breath control, is particularly beneficial in promoting mental calmness and clarity.

7.3. Meditation: Tranquility and Mindfulness

While Yoga largely operates under the purview of physical well-being with aspects of mental peace, Meditation mainly targets our mental well-being, honing our skills of concentration, mindfulness, and inner peace.

7.3.1. Reaping the Mental Benefits of Meditation

Through Meditation, we can manage our stress levels, one of the significant harbingers of many age-related ailments like hypertension, depression, and cognitive decline. Moreover, it cultivates a positive outlook, boosts our memory, and promotes sound sleep, all vital for a rewarding life post 50.

Really, the essence of meditation is mindfulness — the cultivated ability to hold our attention on the present moment non-judgmentally. It allows us to disengage from the constant chatter of our minds, the ruminations about past events, or anxieties about the future, fostering a sense of peace and equanimity.

7.3.2. The Physical Perks of Meditation

Meditation also lends physical advantages, enhancing our immunity and pain tolerance. Regular practice can lead to lower blood pressure and improved digestion, both critical aspects for people over 50. Proven to bring down inflammation, a prevalent issue in age-related diseases, it works wonders for overall longevity.

7.4. The Combined Power of Yoga and Meditation

By combining the potent powers of Yoga and Meditation, we can bridge the divide between our mind and body, all the while improving our total health and quality of life. This synergy is of utmost importance, particularly in our journey of graceful aging–a journey that's not just about adding years to our lives, but life to our years as well!

Remember, the harmonious interplay of Yoga and Mediation builds upon consistent practice. Start slow, respect your body's limitations, and gradually deepen your practices. Seek professional guidance if needed. Make your golden years truly rewarding with these powerful tools, embodying the mantra 'healthy body, sound mind.'

Here's to living life agelessly! Let's keep that vibrancy alive, because age, after all, is just a number.

Chapter 8. Sleep and Rest: The Underrated Wellness Allies

Let's venture into two crucial yet underrated elements of wellness - sleep and rest. As we advance in age, these two aspects become increasingly significant in our health and overall well-being.

8.1. Understanding the Role of Sleep

Firstly, let's delve into sleep, an essential yet often neglected component of health. Sleep is not just about getting a 'shut-eye'; it's a complex process that plays a vital role in various physical and mental functions. Quality sleep offers several benefits, ranging from improved mood and memory to enhanced immunity and longevity.

Deprivation of quality sleep has been associated with an increased risk of chronic conditions such as heart disease, diabetes, obesity and even mental health disorders. It's imperative to respect our body's need for sleep, and prioritize it just as we do for nutrition or physical activity.

8.2. The Aging Sleep

As we cross the 50-year mark, our bodies undergo several changes, and our sleep patterns are no exception. Sleep architecture—the pattern of sleep stages within a certain period—tends to change with age. Older adults might experience a decrease in deep sleep and an increase in lighter sleep stages. They may find it challenging to fall asleep, maintain sleep, or may wake up feeling unrefreshed. It's important to acknowledge these changes and take measures to manage them proactively.

8.3. Cultivating Healthy Sleep Habits

Fortunately, a few simple practices can set the stage for better sleep. Applying proper sleep hygiene—habits that help improve sleep quality—can significantly improve your night's rest. The following are some of the recommended practices:

- Consistent sleep schedule: Maintaining a consistent sleep-wake cycle, even on weekends, can condition your body to a regular sleep pattern. Aim for at least 7 to 9 hours of sleep per night.

- Bedtime rituals: Engage in calming activities before bedtime such as reading, meditating, or having a warm bath. These rituals signal the body that it's time to unwind and prepare for sleep.

- Bedroom environment: Keep your bedroom quiet, dark, and cool. Consider using items such as earplugs, eye shades, a fan, or a noise machine to create an environment conducive to sleep.

- Limit exposure to screens: The light emitted by phones, computers, and TVs can interfere with the body's natural sleep-wake cycle. Limit exposure to these devices close to bedtime.

- Physical activity: Regular exercise can help you fall asleep faster and enjoy deeper sleep.

Remember, consistency is crucial in developing and maintaining good sleep habits. It's not about making dramatic changes overnight but about incremental improvements that, over time, will yield significant results.

8.4. Embracing Rest

Next to sleep, we have its equally important counterpart - rest. Rest is more than the absence of physical activity. It's about allowing our bodies and minds to recover, rejuvenate, and regain balance.

The culture of 'busyness' often dismisses rest as unproductive.

However, science reveals that taking time to rest can boost brain function, foster creativity, increase productivity and even slow the aging process.

8.5. Restorative Techniques

Now let's explore some restorative techniques. You don't necessarily have to sleep or do nothing to rest. Here are a few strategies:

- Mindful meditation: It allows attention to focus on the present moment and promotes relaxation and stress reduction.

- Time in nature: Spending time in green spaces or around nature can reduce stress and promote well-being and relaxation.

- Hobbies: Engaging in activities you enjoy can help you relax and take your mind off stress.

- Breathing exercises: Deep, slow breathing can lower heart rate, reduce anxiety, and promote a sense of calm.

- Progressive muscle relaxation: This technique involves tensing and then releasing different muscle groups to promote physical relaxation.

Remember, there's no one-size-fits-all when it comes to rest. Understanding what refreshes and rejuvenates you is crucial. So experiment with different methods and find your unique 'rest recipe'.

In conclusion, sleep and rest stand as our unsung heroes in the pursuit of wellness. It's high time we give these aspects the importance they deserve in our health regimes. Remember, a rested body is a healthy body, and a well-rested mind contributes to a vibrant life. Embrace the power of good sleep and restful relaxation to ensure age remains just a number for you.

Chapter 9. Mental Fitness: Keeping Your Brain Active and Agile

While physical fitness often steals the spotlight, maintaining mental fitness is equally critical, especially as we edge into our later years. An active, agile mind can significantly contribute to improved overall health and longevity. This chapter dives deep into understanding mental fitness and how we can keep our cognitive faculties agile and robust, even after the half-century mark.

9.1. Understanding Mental Fitness

Just as physical fitness refers to the body's ability to function efficiently, mental fitness is all about your mind's capacity to regain its balance upon disruptions. It's about staying sharp, focused, and able to navigate the complex, ever-changing landscape of life.

Mental fitness involves different mental skills, including attention, focus, recall, critical thinking, creativity, and flexibility. When these skills are maintained or even improved, they can greatly contribute to our quality of life, and significantly reduce the chances of developing neurodegenerative illnesses like Alzheimer's and dementia.

9.2. Why Mental Fitness Matters

The human brain is an intricate, remarkable organ capable of evolving throughout its lifetime. Neuroplasticity is a primary feature that lets the brain alter its structure and functions based on life's experiences. Age can cause the brain's capacity for neuroplasticity to slow down, which is why maintaining mental fitness becomes crucial.

Mental fitness plays a vital role in:

1. Enhancing cognitive reserve: An active brain has a higher cognitive reserve - a buffer against brain disease and age-related cognitive decline.

2. Stress management: Mentally fit individuals cope better with stress, enhancing physical health and lifespan.

3. Emotional well-being: Mental fitness promotes positive thinking, happiness, and resilience.

9.3. The Pillars of Mental Fitness

Several components can play into mental wellness. The following are three critical pillars:

1. Cognitive activities to improve brain function: Activities that stimulate the brain, such as reading, puzzles, or learning new skills.

2. Regular physical exercise aids mental agility: Exercise improves blood flow to the brain and supports cognitive function.

3. A nutritious diet to fuel your brain: Nutrients such as omega-3 fatty acids, antioxidants, and B-vitamins are pivotal for brain health.

9.4. Strengthening the Brain through Cognitive Activities

Challenging the brain with cognitive activities helps boost its health and resilience. Regular engagement in mentally stimulating exercises can substantially improve memory, thinking skills, and problem-solving abilities.

1. **"Puzzles and Board Games:"** Engaging in games that require strategic thinking can be a fun way to stimulate the brain. Chess, Sudoku, crosswords and puzzles are all excellent choices.

2. **"Continuous Learning:"** Remaining a lifelong learner helps the brain form new connections. Consider learning a new language, instrument, or any skill that interests you.

9.5. The Influence of Physical Fitness on Mental Fitness

Engaging in physical exercise isn't just beneficial for the body; it's also pivotal for your brain. Regular workouts increase the flow of blood to the brain, facilitating nutrient delivery and the removal of waste products. It can also improve mood and sleep, and reduce stress and anxiety.

1. **"Aerobic Exercises:"** Activities like walking, running, cycling, or swimming can augment heart rate, improve circulation and enhance brain health.

2. **"Strength Training:"** Weight lifting and resistance training stimulate the nervous system and can slow down cognitive decline.

9.6. Eating for Brain Health

Diet plays an integral role in supporting mental agility. Consuming a nutrient-dense diet helps maintain cognitive functions while protecting against brain diseases.

1. **"Omega-3 Fatty Acids:"** Food sources like fatty fish, walnuts, chia seeds, are rich sources.

2. **"Antioxidants:"** Berries, nuts, green tea, and dark chocolate are chock-full of antioxidants.

3. **"B-Vitamins:"** Whole grains, meat, eggs, and legumes offer an ample supply of this nutrient.

9.7. The Role of Restorative Sleep

Sleep is an underrated ally of mental fitness. During sleep, the body repairs damaged cells, consolidates memories, and primes the mind for optimal functioning the next day. Aim for seven to nine hours of quality sleep each night.

9.8. The Power of Social Interactions

Maintaining social connections can play a significant role in keeping your brain sharp. Being socially active can ward off loneliness and stress that contribute to cognitive decline. Regular interaction with loved ones can stimulate mental activity, fostering a healthier brain.

Age carries its wisdom and, when treated mindfully, our golden years can be a period of growth, happiness, and great mental vitality. By paying attention to mental fitness, we can significantly enhance our lives' quality and embrace the journey of ageless nutrition and fitness with full gusto!

Chapter 10. Managing Chronic Conditions with Nutrition and Exercise

Aging is a natural process accompanied by gradual changes in the body's structure and functions. These alterations can lead to chronic conditions if not carefully managed. Luckily, by understanding the power of nutrition and exercise, we can mitigate these changes and live a healthful, energetic life.

10.1. Understanding Chronic Conditions

Chronic illnesses are long-term medical conditions that require ongoing medical attention and limit daily activities. Notable examples include arthritis, diabetes, heart disease, and Alzheimer's disease, among others. People over 50 are at higher risk due to age-related physiological changes and often require careful management to maintain quality of life. However, with the right nutritional plan and suitable exercise regimen, the risk and impact of these chronic conditions can be significantly reduced.

10.2. Nutrition: Your Anti-aging Arsenal

The quality of food we consume can greatly influence health outcomes. Optimal nutrition can regulate body processes, improve immune function, and slow down aging. Let's delve into some specific dietary habits that can positively affect chronic disease management.

10.2.1. Phytonutrients - Nature's Protectors

Phytonutrients are plant-derived compounds with health-protecting qualities. They reduce inflammation, improve heart health, support immune function, and may help prevent chronic conditions. Eat a rainbow—consume various fruits and vegetables like berries, leafy greens, bell peppers, and sweet potatoes to maximize phytonutrient intake.

10.2.2. Lean Protein - The Building Blocks of Life

Adequate protein intake helps maintain muscle mass, boost immunity, and cardiovascular health. Opt for lean protein sources such as fish, poultry, eggs, legumes, and dairy products, particularly those with lower saturated fats.

10.2.3. Healthy Fats - Long-lasting Energy Stores

Healthy fats support brain health, lower bad LDL cholesterol levels and increase good HDL cholesterol. To leverage these benefits, include avocados, nuts, seeds, olives, and fish in your diet.

10.2.4. Fiber - The Unsung Hero for Gut Health

Dietary fiber improves digestive health, controls blood sugar levels, and helps maintain a healthy weight. Excellent sources include whole grains, fruits, vegetables, nuts, and legumes.

10.3. Exercise: The Elixir of Youth

While proper nutrition lays the foundation, regular physical activity is the cornerstone of managing chronic conditions. Exercise, when tailored to an individual's capacity, can work wonders in enhancing mobility, improving body composition, sustaining mental health, and lessening disease symptoms.

10.3.1. Cardiovascular Exercise for Heart Health

Cardiovascular exercise raises heart rate, promotes lung functionality, and can combat conditions like heart disease and hypertension. Starting slowly with walking, cycling, or swimming can be excellent for beginners.

10.3.2. Resistance Training for Muscular Strength

Resistance or strength training can help maintain lean muscle mass, improve bone density, and manage diseases like arthritis and osteoporosis. You can use resistance bands, weights, or even your body weight for exercises like squats, lunges, or push-ups.

10.3.3. Balance and Flexibility Exercises to Enhance Mobility

Exercises like yoga, tai chi, and Pilates improve balance, prevent falls, and increase flexibility. These are especially beneficial for older adults and can contribute to overall mobility and independence.

10.4. Let's Get Personal: Tailoring Your Health Plan

Remember, the most effective approach to managing chronic conditions is personalized to your individual needs, preferences, and current health status. It's crucial to consult your physician or a trained health professional to determine the optimal nutrient needs and exercise regimen for you.

To sum it up, nutrition, backed by a regulated and suitable exercise regime, forms the key to managing chronic conditions. Embrace a healthful lifestyle to age gracefully - because you're not just adding years to your life, but life to your years.

Chapter 11. Enjoying Life: The Art of Ageless Well-being

At the core of aging is the concept of well-being. There's more to well-being than simply feeling happy or content. It consists of multiple dimensions including physical, emotional, and cognitive well-being, all tied together to create a fulfilling and enjoyable life.

11.1. Physical Well-being

Physical well-being starts with adopting healthy behaviors, like regular physical activity and a balanced diet.

Exercise does more than just help to maintain a healthy weight; it can also improve mental health, increase longevity, and lower the risk of chronic illnesses. People over 50 should aim for a mix of cardio activities, strength training, flexibility exercises, and balance training. It's not about matching the fitness levels of your younger years, but about finding activities that help maintain physical function and prevent illness.

Eating well is equally significant. The body's nutrient needs change as we age, emphasizing certain vitamins, minerals and other components like fiber and healthy fats. A diet filled with fruits, vegetables, lean proteins, whole grains, and low-fat dairy can help meet these needs. Staying hydrated is also paramount, as the sense of thirst diminishes with age.

And let's not forget the importance of sleep. Aging adults should aim for 7 to 9 hours of sleep each night. Quality sleep helps body repair, improves focus and reduces the risk of various health issues.

11.2. Emotional Well-being

Next to physical health is emotional well-being, a cornerstone of overall wellness.

Maintaining social connections can help ensure this. Interacting with loved ones, friends, or community members can fuel feelings of belonging and purpose. It's also crucial to engage in activities that nourish joy, like pursuing a hobby or traveling.

Maintaining a positive attitude is an essential aspect of emotional well-being. This doesn't mean ignoring feelings of sadness or anger, but rather acknowledging them, understanding their source, and finding ways to overcome them. Practicing gratitude can also foster emotional stability by highlighting the good in life.

And never underestimate the value of laughter. It can lower stress, improve mood, and even help mitigate pain.

11.3. Cognitive Well-being

Supporting cognitive health can also promote a sense of well-being while counteracting age-related cognitive decline.

Cognitive stimulating activities, such as puzzles, reading, writing, playing musical instruments, can keep the mind active and fend off cognitive decline. Being a lifelong learner can lead to new skills, open up new vistas, and provide sense of accomplishment.

Another cognitive key is mindfulness. By focusing on the present moment, mindfulness can reduce stress, improve mental function, increase positivity, and enhance relationships.

11.4. Ensuring Ageless Well-being

Aging doesn't have to mean slowing down, losing independence, or surrendering to chronic conditions. It can be a time to flourish, to capitalise on past accomplishments and to embrace new opportunities.

Staying proactive, monitoring your health regularly, staying in touch with your healthcare provider, seeking advice on preventive measures and following recommended screening guidelines are all keys to ensuring a healthy aging process.

Lastly, practicing self-care is invaluable. Whether that means taking a day off to relax, indulging in a beloved activity, or treating yourself to a nutritious meal, these small moments of care can make a significant difference in overall well-being.

In conclusion, age is just a number when it comes to enjoying life. By maintaining a balanced focus on physical, emotional, and cognitive health, you can ensure ageless well-being. No matter how many candles there are on the birthday cake, the passion for life should never flicker. It's not about trying to turn back the clock, but embracing the beauty of the years that have passed, and the many wonderful ones that are yet to come. Age truly is an art, and with this understanding, we can make our golden years vibrantly joyous and fulfilling. Indeed, our life can blossom with age.